DIVA,

I hope you enjoy
this book!

- Jee Q

Weight Loss

D.I.V.A

Discover the Discipline, Inspiration, Victory, and Acceptance within you!

LeeAnn Willis Sims

ISBN: 978-1-4834-2169-8 (sc)
ISBN: 978-1-4834-2170-4 (e)

Library of Congress Control Number: 2014920237

Lulu Publishing Services rev. date: 03/02/2015

Dedication

To everyone young and old, who's fought to find peace with what you see in the mirror. It's time to discover the D.I.V.A. you truly are.

Epigraph

"I've learned by now to be quite content whatever my circumstances. I'm just as happy with little as with much, with much as with little. I've found the recipe for being happy whether full or hungry, hands full or hands empty. Whatever I have, wherever I am, I can make it through anything in the One who makes me who I am."
- Philippians 4:11-13 (The Message)

Contents

Foreword

Many of you can probably relate to looking in the mirror and not liking what you see, or wondering how in the world you ate *all* those chocolate chip cookies. Countless people, myself included, have struggled with weight and how it affects your self-perception and self-acceptance. My very dear friend and mentee, LeeAnn Willis Sims, is no stranger to all of this. Having known her since her childhood, I have witnessed her transformation and growth from a teenager in our church youth group to an extremely polished and accomplished woman. Through the years we have worked together in ministry and in the arts, and she has always been a truly humble, sincere, and hilarious personality, which you will no doubt get a glimpse of as you read through these pages of *Weight Loss D.I.V.A.!*

Weight Loss D.I.V.A. is a very personable and transparent story of LeeAnn's struggle with weight loss and self image. She and I have had many conversations over the years regarding this topic, and even though I am as familiar with her battles as she is with mine, I can honestly say that I was not prepared for the tremendous effect that this book would have on my life. Even as I write this, my eyes are swelling up with tears of happiness, tears of gratefulness, and yes, tears of relief. You see, this book will inspire hope for so many people: the teenager tormented in his or her mind because of the number on the scale, or the woman who feels she will only be happy if she reaches a certain size or looks like a celebrity on television. This book is for the one who doesn't always feel pretty, handsome, or accepted because of weight, which is so many of us!

Finally, I am excited for the mothers and fathers out there who will have a tool that they can share with their teenage sons and daughters to help them navigate through their thoughts and feelings in regards to their own weight and body image. As a mother of two teenage daughters, I regularly tell them how beautiful they are. But I admit that there's just something good about hearing it from someone who doesn't *have* to say these things because they have a vested interest in you. LeeAnn, in a very funny and engaging way, speaks directly to the heart in regards to body image and self-acceptance. I literally laughed out loud several times!

She writes this book as if she's talking to a really close and trusted friend....the friend that says, "Your secret is safe with me". It's personal and relatable, and you easily get the sense that this is someone who cares and understands firsthand what you are going through. As I read, I pictured acting auditions I've attended where men and women (myself included!) have stood outside pulling, tugging, and stretching out clothes while sucking in their stomachs and sizing up everyone else in the room. It's so exhausting! But this book, *Weight Loss D.I.V.A.*, offers a beautiful, refreshing approach and reminder to how I need to see myself.

So, whether you are a size two or a size twenty-two, the words on the pages of this book speak loudly to the person who is striving endlessly to be in love with the beautiful person that they already are. Thank you, LeeAnn Willis Sims.

- Marcia Myers

Acknowledgments

To my husband Michael, I am so much better with you. Thank you for your partnership, strength, and love. To my dad, thank you for loving me the way only a father could and passing on your gift to write. To my mom, thank you for signing me up for that makeover and believing in me before I had the courage to believe in myself. To my family and closest friends, thank you for seeing me beyond my exterior and treating me just the same no matter what my size. To my coaches along the way including Amanda, Beverly, Chuck, Marcia, and Terri, thank you for pushing me hard, ignoring my whining, and making me tougher. To my editor, Christina, thank you for taking on this project as if it were your own. To my Pastors, thank you for the much needed moments of inspiration that reminded me of the strength I have in Christ. Above all, I thank my Lord and Savior, Jesus Christ, for accepting me just the way that I am and loving me in a way that I may never fully understand.

Introduction

Being skinny is not all it's cracked up to be.

When I was a little girl, I had dreams of being thin. As early as the fifth grade, I was aware of being overweight and instinctively knew that to be successful in this world, you had to be thin. I thought everything would be perfect, that *I* would be perfect, once I was thin. It was in the fifth grade that boys and girls split up in health class to learn about the beauty of puberty by an outdated video of course. In the back of the classroom I sat with my legs crossed, listening intently to the narrator as he said, "some girls gain weight when they begin to menstruate, and some may lose weight." Silently, I said to myself, *I want to be one of the girls who loses weight.* It was also in the fifth grade that I stood on the scale in the nurse's office weighing in at a solid 150 pounds. She sent a note of concern home to my mother and told me that if I just stayed at that weight (forever) I would grow up to be a healthy adult. *Are you serious?? How can you expect an already chubby kid to not gain an ounce over the next fifteen years?*

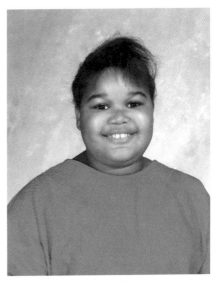

That's me in elementary school . . . don't you just want to pinch those cheeks?!

For me, being thin was not an option. I have diaries full of other dreams, like marriage, children, and acting on Broadway. Yet, all of the mental images of my future included a "thin" LeeAnn, not the one I saw in real life at 289 pounds. Losing weight seemed to be the key to success in my life and the only way to start my life's journey. And finally, in the year 2008, I achieved that goal.

I started this book four or five years ago, as I was nearing the end of a very successful weight loss plan. By the beginning of 2008 I boasted a 144-pound weight loss. I was on top of the world and featured in some national magazines and even on "The Today Show" for my accomplishment. Everywhere I went people who knew the larger version of me asked how I lost the weight. Quite honestly, I didn't have just one perfect way to lose it. I started a few years before that on a protein shake and supplement diet; then focused on holistic health with many vegetarian options; and then ended with another meal-replacement plan that helped me drop the last set of pounds. Slowly but surely, I changed my life. I was so proud that I had finally accomplished a childhood dream—to be thin! I wanted to share what I learned with the world. After years of dieting and weight loss plans, I had realized that it took much more than just eating well to lose a substantial amount of weight.

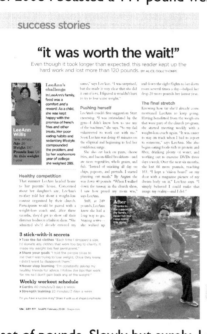

Although I had tons of diet and exercise tips to share, the best tip of all is this: *Being thin does not equal happiness.* For a skinny person, this may seem like an obvious fact, but it is not so obvious for people who've struggled with their weight. When I finally reached the size I always wanted to be, I realized that I was not satisfied. I still had insecurities about my body and began to focus on other characteristics about myself that appeared to be lacking.

Years later, I am nearly back to the weight at which I started my journey. I'm not as cheery as I used to be, and sometimes I honestly doubt whether or not I can lose the weight again. So this book is as much for me as it is for you. I'm reminded that being successful does not mean you have a perfect story. It means you just don't give up. If I had released this book in 2008, it would have sold a ton of copies—"Hear tips from a weight loss success story!" But that's no longer my platform. Instead, I encourage you to join me on this journey to rediscover (or discover for the first time) the strength that's within us to achieve our dreams.

Yes, weight loss success takes more than eating salads and becoming a gym rat! I've learned that it's about Discipline (physical, mental, and spiritual); seeking Inspiration; walking in Victory; and Accepting yourself, no matter what. That's what being a "Weight Loss D.I.V.A." is all about. In this book, I will reflect on a few lessons I've learned along the way that helped me lose half of my size, and that will hopefully help *you* to rediscover the D.I.V.A. within.

LeeAnn

Chapter I

Discipline

Summer 2001

Looking back at the moment I started my weight loss journey, I can still remember my excitement. I could only imagine the possibilities that were ahead...finally being thin! After two months on my first diet program, I thought I was doing pretty well. And one of the greatest confidence boosters was the attention I received. People were finally starting to notice the changes in my body. I kept thinking to myself, *Don't mess this thing up.* My commitment amazed even myself; my work was actually paying off! Recently I even mustered up enough courage to turn down a home-cooked family dinner so I could stick to my weight loss plan. I don't know how I did it, but I actually sat at the dinner table with my family and chugged my protein shake while they indulged in macaroni 'n cheese, fried chicken, and buttery rolls.

There is *no* way I could have said "no" to all this yummy food before. But at the start of my weight loss journey, it was as if something finally clicked in me. It dawned on me—I want this more than I've wanted anything at this point. That initial vision and hope pushed me through some of the hardest times and gave me the courage I needed to make the really tough decisions, like eating out and handling big family dinners.

Despite this initial surge of determination, I faced a huge obstacle that summer, a family reunion in Georgia. I had to admit that I was nervous, and I knew preparation was key to not falling off the wagon. First things first, I told myself, as I studied the schedule of activities and planned my meals accordingly. I packed my shakes in sandwich bags to ration out my meals for the day. Knowing that everyone else would be eating fast food during the car ride from Philadelphia, I also brought lots of healthy snacks like carrot sticks and apples to keep me on track. We arrived, and I survived without falling off my diet. I patted myself on the back. Day one of the reunion went off without a hitch, and I was proud of myself.

The next morning I toured the "city" of Americus (only a few blocks long) with my family. Then we headed to the mecca of the South for lunch—Waffle House. This didn't bother me one bit, though. I had practiced resisting fattening foods for the last two months of my diet, and I had become somewhat of a pro at sticking to my plan. While everyone else was eating waffles, greasy fried chicken, and hamburgers with French fries, I had a grilled chicken salad made to order. *This establishment is clearly not famous for its healthy menu options*, I thought, as I looked down at my plate. My salad looked like they took the lettuce right off a hamburger bun, slapped it onto my plate, and threw a piece of chicken on top with mayo and ketchup as the dressing. Yet surprisingly, I didn't care. I was focused. Another successful day down. This reunion was a breeze, or so I thought.

Although we were supposed to be done with the activities for the evening, my grandfather wanted to have dinner with us at one of his favorite places. Everyone else was hungry again and quickly agreed with the change of plans. Enter my greatest opponent thus far: the buffet.

I mean, who was really going to turn down "all you can eat" food? Within seconds I began to panic—clearly, this meal was not in my plan. How was I going to pull this one off? My mind scrolled back to previous victories. When faced with this situation a few weeks ago at the family dinner, I just stood my ground and drank my shake at the table with everyone else. But this was different. We were actually going *out* to eat. How could I bring my shake to dinner? Could I resist all that food? And did I mention this was not in the plan???

My thoughts instantly started raging within me. *This is ridiculous! This is so silly! Why does eating healthy have to be so difficult?* The truth is I wasn't even hungry. I was just embarrassed, and I didn't want my newly acquainted relatives to notice. My immediate family knew about my weight loss plan, and that was enough, as far as I was concerned. Furthermore, I didn't want to explain myself or my diet to every last family member there. All I wanted was to blend in and just be "normal."

This may sound dramatic (and it is), but when I walked into the restaurant that evening, everything seemed to be in slow motion. My stomach was in knots. I felt so nervous, and yet, still somewhat prepared. I rehearsed my game plan for the meal: sit quietly at the table, act like nothing is wrong, and watch everyone eat while enjoying a delicious glass of water or a Diet Coke. Okay, not the best plan I know, but a plan nonetheless. Before I could even take a seat, my eyes rested on the lanes of food staring at me, waiting for me, challenging me.

I froze.

This time, I couldn't be courageous. I couldn't sit at the table and watch everybody eat like I did a few weeks before. I couldn't face my fear and just suck it up while everybody else was having fun. I had to leave. Fighting back the tears, I pulled my cousin to the side and politely asked her to drive me back to the motel. We hopped in her car without me doing so much as to say goodbye to anyone. Once we reached the car, I finally let the tears fall as we rode back in silence. I cried the entire way to the motel.

When I returned to my room, I was so angry. I couldn't believe I had run away! Once again, this diet was keeping me from enjoying myself, and I felt like I couldn't do anything about it. I sulked in the room for a while by myself with the shades pulled down and the room dark and quiet. I felt so alone. No one was around. It was just me.

Then, something clicked. I had to do something. I needed to gain back control.

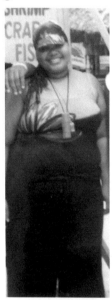

In my frustration, I put on my one-piece bathing suit with the ugly blue flower, capri pajama pants, white sweat socks and sneakers. With utter resolve, I headed for the motel gym. I could not let this thing defeat me. While everyone was at the buffet getting their grub on, I decided to fight the thing that had me feeling like crap. It was my way of responding. I felt like the weight was literally beating me down, but it was my turn to get in a few punches.

The gym was extremely small, just like the town. There was a twelve-inch 1980s-style television mounted in the center of the room, a shelf with rolled-up white towels, a stationary bike, a few weight machines, and (my all time

Just in case you didn't believe me—I really did wear that ugly bathing suit and capri pants . . . favorite) a treadmill. It was one of those old-school manual, motor-less treadmills. You know the one you have to walk on to actually make it move? It made squeaky noises with every step. I walked on that thing as if each step were my last. Pumping my arms hard, I fought against the

obstacles that had confronted me for so long. I increased my speed and intensity with every tear that tried to trickle down my face, repeating to myself, "I am going to beat this thing."

About three-quarters of the way into my workout, my uncle came to check on me. He entered the room, and with a smile as big as day and his voice as loud as can be, said, "That's my niece, go 'head girl!" That's all it took for me to keep going. His one comment was enough for me to know that I had made the right decision.

Soon after my aunt joined us, followed by others who came to see what was going on. It was as if the party came to me. We joked, they made me laugh, and I finished my day without compromising my decision to get healthier.

That brief weekend in Georgia taught me so much about weight loss, determination, and discipline. Once again, my diet had me feeling trapped in a box, alone again. Only this time, I couldn't seem to fight my way out. I was so angry and frustrated because I felt like I was not in control of the situation. My plan for the day was not working, and I did not have an immediate alternative. It was like the annoyance you experienced as a child when the bigger kids played "keep-away" with your ball. The plan was mine, but someone else had gained control of it. I couldn't stay at the motel alone because my family would try to make me come with them. On the other hand, I couldn't drink a protein shake at the buffet—that just looks stupid. So despite my apprehension and lack of ideal choices, I went to the restaurant anyway, only to leave a short while later.

Much to my surprise, no one chastised me for leaving dinner early that day. I realized that I could not expect the world to stop and consult my plans before changing. That just isn't realistic or fair. I had to make the situation work for me, meaning that sometimes I may have to experience uncomfortable circumstances. But I also learned that the discomfort only lasts a little while. Sometimes I have to make tough choices and re-prioritize my life. And other times I will have to stand alone. I learned that eating well or exercising does not mean loving my family or the things I like to do any less. It just means I may have to enjoy them in a different way. That day, I loved my family *and* enjoyed their company, but I also put myself first. Expressing love towards them didn't have to mean eating junk food along with them; I could still enjoy their time, just not necessarily at a place that jeopardized the achievement of my personal goals. I made my commitment to being healthy more important than spending an hour at a buffet laughing and eating with those I loved. Instead, I endured a tough workout and still had the opportunity to be with them later.

To me, discipline is more about adopting a certain way of thinking and doing, rather than self-inflicted punishment or always eating perfectly. Just like in Leslie, Georgia, I'm faced with the same decisions today. And, I wish I could say I always make the so-called "right" choice. But I don't. I don't always eat the way I know I should to lose weight and keep the pounds off; I don't always exercise; and sometimes, I just feel like moping around and indulging in a big dose of self-pity. Sometimes I don't feel strong—actually most of the time, I don't feel strong. But you know what? Discipline is not always doing the "disciplined" thing; discipline is consistently getting back up.

Discipline is not always doing the "disciplined" thing; discipline is consistently getting back up.

This type of discipline is one of the most important life lessons, and probably one of the most difficult to master. From my experience, I've found that you only learn to get back up through training and practice. Doing the same thing over and over can drive you crazy, but in this case, it's absolutely necessary for your physical and mental well-being. I have to train my mind to NOT fall into depression when I don't stick to the plan exactly. And I have to practice forgiving myself when I've gained some weight. So what about the four slices of pizza you devoured last night? Yes, it will take training and discipline to get you to the gym! But above all, I have to train myself to believe that I am beautiful and perfect *today*—without losing another pound and without having abs of steel. In this moment, I'm just as great as I will ever be.

I want you to understand how much I can relate to the struggles you may be facing. Today as I write, I sit here just a few pounds shy of where I started. I realize I'm the statistic that "gained it all back." Wow! Even admitting that in writing is mind-blowing. Yet if I were to focus on that fact every single day and every single time I looked in the mirror, I could never win again. And maybe, just maybe, I am happy as I am now. All I need to do is recognize that I want to lose weight and decide to work towards my goal. But I can't spend my days mourning the weight loss of my past. Truthfully, I don't know how I've gained all that weight back. And, yes, I am disappointed that I did. But, I'm here today, and all I can do is work on changing today.

Now we all know this is easier said than done. Becoming disciplined is going to take patience (with yourself, most of all!), determination, and focused energy. However, the results are truly life-changing! At this moment you may be wringing your hands in frustration because of past failed attempts. Trust me; I've been there, especially with dieting. Diets can serve as a big roadblock for those of us who have struggled with our weight because we tend to not stick to them. And unfortunately, once we get on the scale and see that we've gained a few pounds back we fall all the way off the wagon and have to start the cycle all over again. This is crazy! Once I realized that it was left up to me to manage my weight loss journey, I started to hold myself more accountable to my goal – but even that wasn't easy.

Think about it, here I was a person who had been conditioned to eat whatever I wanted whenever I wanted it, all the way going back to when I was a little girl. So how in the world was I going to "deprogram" myself? In my mind being disciplined like this seemed so restrictive; I saw it as a self-imposed prison. So not only was I battling the weight, but also my thinking in an area I had never wanted to touch – self-discipline in my eating habits.

For me, discipline even went beyond the struggles of healthy eating. For years food had comforted and soothed me, and in time had become one of my best friends. Food helped me to feel better about myself and my situation, even though it was a fleeting feeling. Adopting healthier eating habits posed a definite threat to that feeling of gratification and comfort. Plain and simple, discipline seemed like a punishment, and who likes to be punished? You must admit, you probably experience an initial gut-reaction when we hear the term. For some of us, the word triggers childhood memories of time-outs and spankings, or perhaps adult realities of sitting in a gray cubicle for eight hours day after day. For me, discipline meant doing something I hated to do in order to get something I would love to have. Boy was I wrong! Discipline is not self-hatred or a form of self-punishment, but actually an expression of the love you have for yourself. When you love someone, you do what's best for them, right? It took me years to come to this realization. I had always seen discipline as taking away, instead of giving back to myself. I forced down foods I didn't really like and turned away those I thoroughly enjoyed; I also made myself clock countless hours in the gym for unimaginative workouts that left me sore, sweaty, and bored out of my mind.

Through dieting, I wanted to punish the "fat" so it would never want to come back again. I hated it. Yet, I now realize that I could never separate the "fat" from me. For better or for worse, it was a part of who I was. So, instead of just punishing the fat, I was actually punishing myself. Although I was engaged in healthy activities meant to build myself up, the driving force behind it was actually self-destructive. I never wanted to see the "me" I knew again. I did not like what I had become, and dieting became my only way out. Discipline gradually evolved into an act of self-hatred and for that reason, I hated dieting.

But once I started doing the little things like exercising and turning down that Popeyes chicken, I began to see that there are benefits to discipline—the extra energy, added confidence, and overall sense of pride from making better food choices. I had to remember that I was doing this for me. Losing weight can't just be about looking good or squeezing into jeans you never imagined you could fit into. One of the most important aspects of weight loss is HEALTH. Let me say that again, you have to remember that becoming healthier is one of the main benefits of shedding unwanted weight. Although I am relatively young, many young overweight people suffer from diseases like hypertension, diabetes, joint problems, and the beginning signs of heart disease. So in order to avoid these in my life, I had to begin to see the overall health benefit of losing weight in a new light.

Sometimes it *can* be overwhelming, you know. But you can't stress yourself out about all the work you have to do or all the pounds you want to lose. Now that I am in a position where I am pursuing total wellness and not just a thinner frame, my approach to losing weight has changed. Although I've been able to shed pounds quickly in the past, I'd rather not speed through the process, because experience has taught me that wellness begins in the heart and mind. More importantly, as I said before I've discovered that being skinny does not equal happiness.

When I first started gaining weight, I remember looking at myself in the mirror and complaining about how much bigger I looked at ten pounds over my goal weight. Today I wish I were only that big! I realize that my discontentment at each step made it difficult to see how fabulous I actually was. Ironically, "perfect" for me right now would be the imperfect size I was back then. I regret the moments I did not enjoy as a thinner woman, and I promised myself I would do things differently this time. We all need to appreciate each step of the journey, no matter what the scale says.

And for each step, I believe that there is peace available to you. It is possible to lose weight without the added pressure of having to accomplish it *right now*. Certain actions can help you to slow down and work towards lasting weight loss success. If you're like me, for example, you've put yourself on strict and structured plans for short bursts of time without uncovering *why* you are even overweight in the first place. Try answering these questions the next time you find yourself staring into a pint of Ben and Jerry's or a huge pepperoni pizza: Are you self-medicating because of that bad breakup? Is this your stress reliever after a long day of work?

Do you celebrate every milestone with a large pizza? Or have you always been the non-athletic "big kid" and don't even know why you eat so much?

I can answer "yes" to all of these questions at some point. But as I took the time to address these issues, I had greater control over the choices I made that would lead to better health *and* a slimmer waistline. Although it has been difficult to take things slowly, I'm willing to wait for what I want, knowing that it will bring lasting results.

Chapter 2

Inspiration

Spring 2008

Now that I had become determined to turn my health around, I had to put my newfound discipline into action. Not one to do anything half way, I decided to sign up for an exercise boot camp. Boot camp was something unlike anything I had ever tried before physically. And given the fact that a former NFL player trained us, it was probably the most challenging physical activity I had ever set out to do. But it was such a fulfilling experience. The great part about being in this boot camp was the location, only about ten minutes from my house. The bad part though was the starting time—5:30 a.m.! That meant a 5:15 arrival time, which also meant waking up at 4:45 five days a week! And, there was no such thing as being late . . . if you weren't on the field with your exercise mat in tow at 5:30; everyone had to do extra jumping jacks or push-ups in your honor. Chuck Morris, a fellow church member and the head trainer, saw to this. He brought intense energy and made sure we brought our best to each session. He was (and still is) insane! The moment I realized this was my first week of boot camp.

The alarm went off at 4:45 a.m. "Urggghhhh," I said, putting the clock on snooze for a bit more sleep. My alarm sounded once again before the crack of dawn reared its ugly head. It's time for boot camp. It had only been a few days so far, but I had to admit I was enjoying it. The people were great, Chuck was a riot, and I was getting an amazing workout—an amazingly difficult workout five days a week to be exact. The only downside? I hated waking up so early. My routine involved slamming the snooze button a few times, punching my pillows, and making numerous proclamations of how much "I don't-wanna-goooooo!" in my whiniest voice before my feet even hit the carpet of my bedroom.

Wait a minute — listen to that beautiful sound. Rain! I smiled smugly to myself, knowing that boot camp would be cancelled. Surely we couldn't exercise in the rain. But just to be sure I could duck back under my covers guilt-free, I checked the camp's blog for a cancellation announcement—I saw nothing. There can't be boot camp today, can there? I'll just go to the track and check it out. I'd feel good knowing that at least I *tried* to workout, and I could go back to sleep in peace.

As I pulled up, there weren't too many cars around. The only sign of life as far as I could see was the lonely street light shining on the puddles in the parking lot. *There's no way we're having boot camp today. I'm sure Chuck will cancel it,* I thought hopefully. Not! I looked over, and yup, there he was. I can't believe he's here. It's pouring outside. This is crazy! Or, maybe I'm crazy for being out here!

With my water bottle and towel in hand, I joined the rest of my "battle buddies" on the track. Much to my surprise, I wasn't the only crazy boot-camper on the field. Actually there were about fifteen of us out there, in the dark, and in the rain at 5:30 in the morning. We all shared the same half-confused look on our faces. One of the coaches started passing out ponchos, as if that were really going to keep us from getting wet. The brim of my hat was the only thing that stood between me and the rain falling on my face.

What was I doing out here? What about my hair? (And let all the black girls say "Amen!").

My mind was racing wondering why I even decided to go through with this. Why in my right mind would I leave my house in the rain when I knew boot camp was held in the middle of a football field? Maybe I really *was* crazy....

Chuck was as loud and energetic as any other normal, dry day. "Jog in place!" he ordered. *Jog in place? Where were we going? Shouldn't he have let us go home by now? Squats. Jogging in place. Squats. What in the world were we doing??*

But about halfway into the workout I realized something: I had forgotten that I wasn't *supposed* to be working out in the rain. Squats. Jogging in place. Squats. Leg raises. Who knew? Was this the new normal? My trainer gave us a pep talk, for which he is now famous: "You are no longer mere mortals. Your reality has now changed." And, it certainly had. Just a few weeks before this, I would have never been caught in the rain doing anything besides running to or from my car, and I *definitely* would not be working out. My reality had changed.

The bar was raised that day. Physically, it wasn't all that hard, but the mental challenge to ignore my surroundings was the toughest experience I had up to that point. Look, I'm not an athlete. I never experienced playing field hockey or soccer in the rain, or having a coach bark orders in my ear—I was just me. But that day, I changed. This was a new me.

Clearly, getting through boot camp that first time was a big step. But staying committed to it for the long haul was a leap. Soon after starting my second eight-week session, I hit a wall. My endurance and self-confidence had increased, but the number on the scale refused to budge. I'll be honest with you. I knew I had not been very strict with the prescribed eating program the second time around. I had reached a point where I literally felt like my diet was out of control. In fact, it seemed as if my cravings were the ones in the driver's seat. Fast food became the norm, yet brought little satisfaction. For two weeks straight I ate fried or fast food every night after work, not counting the restaurant outings and mom's Sunday dinner on the weekend. The scary part is I did not know how to regain control. For a couple days I would eat healthier and feel my stomach going down. But, I would quickly get back on the "junk food wagon."

My exercise routine also took a hit. Even though I worked out hard, I didn't attend regularly or push myself to do something extra on my off days. As the last weigh-in approached, each camp member had to face the scale one final time. So, here I was... Judgment Day, and my turn to jump on the scale. I knew that I had probably not lost any weight, but I was not at all prepared for what I was about to see – 187 pounds?

No, check that again, I thought to myself, *that can't be right.* But, it was. Instead of losing weight, I had gained weight. I moved over to the next station to measure my body fat percentage, desperately hoping that I could at least boast a reduction in that area: 33%. *Thirty-three percent?* While I tried to laugh it off in front of my trainers, I was devastated and terrified. Fear and shame began to cloud my thinking: *I'm almost at 190, which means I'm almost back up to 200. How could I have gained weight and two percentage points of body fat after working out like a dog for two months?! How could this happen?* I ran to my car to pick up the signed copy of the *Essence Magazine* I'd promised my trainer. The note read, "Thanks for helping me stay 'fit and fab!'"

Please.

I was not "fit" or "fab." I was actually quite obese, or felt like it anyway.

I could barely look anyone in the face for the rest of camp. We took pictures and congratulated each other for finishing. Although I was smiling on the outside, I felt like I had not accomplished anything. I was just going through the motions. *What's wrong with me*, I asked myself. *If I tell people so often that "any diet program will work for you if you just work the diet," why is my own advice not working for me anymore?* I had no idea.

By the time I pulled into my driveway from boot camp that morning, my eyes were filled with tears. Fearful thoughts came pouring in, as well as an overwhelming sense of disappointment in the "role model" I was supposed to be. My mind kept replaying my trainer's reaction when she looked at the scale and then at me. She didn't need to say anything—we both knew what I was thinking. Even sitting there afterwards, I could not believe I had messed up (again). I had worked so hard to lose weight, only to regain it back! I would not; I could not go back. I just couldn't! *I can't be a statistic,* I thought. *People are watching; everyone is watching.* But I didn't know how to keep the weight off. That same discipline that I had before when I first started my weight loss journey had vanished somehow. I didn't have it anymore, or I couldn't find it to tap into it. All I saw was the number "200" on the scale, haunting me. It seemed inevitable that I would gain most of the weight back. It was time to ask myself some difficult questions—Why was I back here again? What was the real issue behind all of this? I sat in my car for the next five minutes, tears streaming down my face, and cried out to God, "HELP!!!!!"

Have you ever been there before? I'm sure you've had a moment like this when you were short on inspiration. You know, when you're at the end of your rope and you need a little help beyond yourself? When I was at my lowest point in that car, I needed something bigger and stronger to get me over the hump. That simple prayer inspired me because it reminded me that I did not have to do it alone. Inspiration is anything outside of yourself that reminds you of the bigger picture and sparks motivation to pursue your goals. The secret about inspiration is that it is divinely ignited through God. Anything around us can inspire us. When you have the right attitude, you will begin to see inspiration in the smallest things. For instance, seeing someone like me sweating it out at the gym or hearing another person's success story motivates me.

I get a lot of inspiration through music too. You could be riding in your car feeling a bit down because you ate all those French fries for lunch by yourself. Then suddenly "It's a New Day" by Will.I.Am.

comes on the radio, and it could be just what you need to get back on track. The point is, start looking for inspiration all around you. Look for it at work, church, home, school or just out and about. Trust me; inspiration is something we all can find because it's around us all the time.

Here's my "dream board." I posted it to the back of my bedroom door so that I'd be forced to stare at it each time I leave the house. Although I took it down once I reached my goal the first time, I put it back up now that I'm working towards becoming healthier again. In fact, now I have three boards plastered around my room.

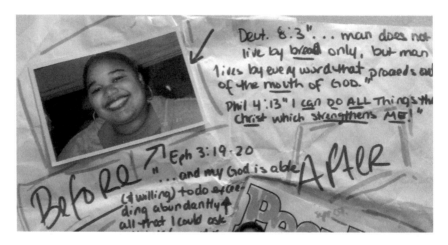

Not only is inspiration all around us, but it also carries a lot of power with it to drive out fear. Fear can't exist when inspiration is present. Why is this? Simply put, inspiration comes from focusing on the positive, while fear emphasizes the negative. Fear bullied me onto a path of gaining all the weight back that I lost. Although I wanted to be thin, I feared what would happen once I did. I was afraid that I might turn into someone I did not want to be—the *health nut*, the *gym freak*, or even worse *the statistic*. My eyes were so fixed on what *could* happen that I soon retreated to my comfort zone where I felt safe. Somehow I rationalized, "If I do not *try* to succeed, I cannot fail to succeed." The more you focus on what you're afraid of, the scarier the monster becomes. So be purposeful in looking for the good around you, and keep your eyes in that direction. Instead of the number on the scale, think on how much easier it will be to walk or run, or how great it will feel to fit into that new dress. Focus on the benefits of a longer life. This is vital because ultimately fear paralyzes you and hinders you from even making that first step towards your goal. That's why gaining courage through inspiration is so important. Looking back, enrolling in boot camp inspired me, though I faced difficulties along the way. Overall, to see myself becoming stronger and healthier was what I needed to give me inspiration to keep going and not give up, no matter how tired I was.

And it doesn't stop there. Inspiration will also give you hope, and who doesn't need that? Without hope what is there to live for? No matter how dark it may look, as long as you have a glimmer of hope, you are on track to achieve your dreams. It's important to get through those dark moments on your journey and to keep moving forward. It's never too late to start over if and when you do fall off the wagon. Whatever you do, just keep going and that motivation will overtake any negative feelings you may be having at the moment.

Speaking of "falling off the wagon," let's take time to have a reality check. We are all human and make mistakes, so don't condemn yourself when you do slip back into old habits. You may have spent your whole life practicing bad habits, so it will take some time to do just the opposite—to become healthier. Each goal you attain should give you inspiration to achieve another goal. For example, as I started working out more I started to see the weight come off. The first twenty pounds were great, but they also motivated me to see the next twenty come off. Each goal I achieved brought me closer to the next one. As long as you have breath in your body, you will always be revising your goals. Sure, you'll have moments where it seems like nothing is happening, but if you remain consistent you *will* achieve them!

This really hits home for me. I remember a time when I felt bad about being fat and not being motivated to lose the weight. Now, you may know women who accept and own their fatness and are even proud of it, but that just wasn't me. I wasn't proud of the fact that I couldn't shop at regular stores or get the finest guy in the room. I honestly felt like something was wrong with me if I didn't lose weight.

And it didn't help that my size made me stick out like a sore thumb, or so I thought. I always felt different from everybody else. On top of that, I took great care not to hang around a lot of "big" girls or do the "watch out for the big girl" dance at parties because I felt like that would bring more attention to *my* problem. Crazy, right? I know it's totally abnormal to think this way, but I thought that if "we" split up, we could go so much further in our goal of fitting in (Please don't tell me I'm the only one who's done this LOL). The sad part is, even when others did accept me as a friend, I still didn't feel like I fit in. I mistakenly thought that everything else about me was perfect, and being overweight was the only thing standing in between me and "normal" (whatever that is!).

But, to my surprise, skinny doesn't equal normal or perfection. We're all oddly imperfect in our own right! That's why for me, losing weight had to stop being about fitting in with the crowd per se. That would never completely happen. I had to make it about my overall health – mentally, physically and spiritually. When you keep the focus off of everyone else and do it for yourself, you'll be amazed at the results and satisfaction. And looking for sources of inspiration by focusing on what really matters—like your overall health—will keep you motivated and will help you reach your goal.

Chapter 3

Victory

Spring 2008

When you keep your eyes on your own goals, define your own success, and consider your own journey to be unique, every little win can turn into a victory. During boot camp I experienced this firsthand. By that year I was getting better at applying discipline to my food and exercise habits, and doing my best to remain inspired and not give up on myself. But soon after joining the program I faced the biggest test thus far—a 5k race. Keep in mind, before I started the weight loss process, I couldn't run more than a few minutes without being totally out of breath. And now I was attempting to run over three miles! Sure, I had dreamed about running a race, but never thought I'd actually *do* it (or didn't know *when* I'd actually do it!).

You know, things have a way of not always working out as planned. When I first signed up for boot camp my intention was to lose some weight. That was a big enough goal in itself! At the start of the program our trainers told us that we could either take the runner's route and prepare for a 5k race, or do martial arts and work up to a yellow belt. I honestly was not in a rush to do either. Couldn't we just do some pushups, run around the track, and call it a day? I had to make a decision. Although the idea was scary, I chose the running route. Of course, I assumed that we'd do it at the *end* of the camp—a comfortable two months later. I knew I could be in shape to run the race by then.

But, God had another plan.

One day the camp owner interrupted one of our workout sessions. With a stack of papers in his arms, he invited us to fill out forms for the imminent race. Then, with a "by the way" attitude, he dropped a bomb on us. Imagine my surprise when I realized I would be running the 5k in the fourth week! And I didn't find out until the third week! Talk about no time to mentally prepare. However, at that time, I had a choice. I could decline the invitation, or step up to the plate and do the race. With fear and trembling, I said I would go through with it.

That being said, one week clearly did not allow for much training and preparation. We hit the ground running though, with weekly exercises to build our endurance. Our running coach, Ray, was a friendly guy from Brooklyn who had accepted the challenge to whip us into shape. Thankfully, he exercised a great deal of patience with us, even as he shared his vast knowledge of running and kept us entertained with his stories.

To my amazement, the first Saturday training session wasn't that awful. Ray took it easy on us, grouping us together as we ran around the track at a moderate pace. "Stick together!" he yelled, "Jog the straights, walk the curves!" As we were running, I tried to keep pace with him at the front of the pack. Although I was by no means the fastest person, I did not want to be caught last for the sake of my own personal competitiveness and pride.

Yet by far the greatest challenge for me was maintaining a steady breath. I had heard that the key with running any race is to find the right pace. If you start out too fast, you will be ready to give up halfway through the race. I struggled through each lap, trying to catch my breath. "How. . .[gasp]. . .am I. . .[gasp]. . .supposed. . .to breathe?" I asked Ray in between uncontrolled breaths. He explained that I needed to find my own personal rhythm. Relax my shoulders and arms, he said, and just let my legs do the work. To keep me from tensing up, he also encouraged me to keep my thumbs in-between my index and middle fingers. This actually worked. I jogged three steps while breathing in, and jogged another three while breathing out. I kept the same rhythm even while walking. My goal was not to learn *how* to run, but just to keep breathing steadily. It didn't come overnight though; in fact, it probably took me a few Saturdays to get this rhythm down pat. Soon enough, I could run an entire quarter of a mile without stopping. I don't know about you, but this was a huge accomplishment for the girl who could barely walk a mile in an hour a few years ago. Eventually, the class graduated from the track and took it to the streets. We jogged up and down the hills of Willingboro, New Jersey, sometimes a mile, sometimes six with multiple breaks. We became a family where no one was left behind.

When the trainers announced the quickly approaching 5k run, a measure of fear shot through my chest. Maybe you can relate. Even with all the training or preparation in the world, fear sometimes rises up when it comes time to perform. For me, the idea of completing a race was staggering. How could I run three miles without stopping? Without taking too much time to think about it, I just signed up anyway. Besides, I reasoned, the whole camp was in this together.

I was determined to be in the best shape possible, and was willing to push myself to accomplish this dream of crossing the finish line. You could say that this was my inspiration. The week before the race, I headed to the track on my own. I had heard that if I could run two miles, I could certainly run three on game day. Being the non-athletic girl in the family and in many of my social circles, I wanted to reinvent myself. Before I would have never considered myself an athlete or a runner, but now I was.

The days leading up to the race passed quickly, and suddenly it was the night before the big day. My best friend and I traded some laughs and stories over pasta. I didn't want to stay out too late, but I couldn't contain my enthusiasm. I felt brand new. I told her about the race and how excited I was to complete it the next day. I could tell she was proud of me. With her support and my newfound confidence, I knew that I could do it.

The next morning, I woke up early and headed to the race location, a high school about fifteen minutes from my house. It turned out to be a major community event, with proceeds going to breast cancer research. Students and members from the area gathered around to cheer us along. First I jogged a lap to warm up then positioned myself to take off. Imagine this—hundreds of jittery teenagers and other supporters surrounded the track like a glorified tailgate with their tents, barbecue grill stations, and megaphones. There was also a large stage set up where a band plucked a few chords for their sound check. A gigantic digital clock was placed on either side of the starting line. Finally, the gun went off and it was time to go!

As I began to run, I remembered Ray's advice on keeping a steady pace: find your own rhythm. I ended up running much slower than some others on the track, but I couldn't care less. I was in the zone. I found myself jogging in tandem with another camper who had caught up. Although some had sped past me in the beginning, I later looked back to realize that my slow and steady approach had me ahead of those same quick-footed people. I was tired, but felt re-energized each time I passed a section of students who cheered me on with high-fives

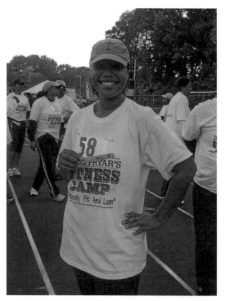

That's me at the finish line. You can't see it, but the popsicle stick indicates my race time— 41.17—good for a first timer!

and pom-poms. It was a physical and mental push, but with everything in me, I made myself keep running. I can't describe how proud I was when I finally crossed that finish line – I did it!

This experience showed me a lot of things. Running a race is not much different than setting out and finishing anything in life. The key is to find your pace. Always remember that only *you* will be the one to finish this race called weight loss. Look at it more as a marathon and not a quick sprint. You didn't get to the size you are overnight, so taking the weight off will require some patience and steadfastness on your part.

Think about it this way—the fact that you are even *trying* to improve your well-being puts you ahead of the pack already. Participating in the 5k taught me that.

But I had to remind myself that it's the small wins over time that build into greater victories.

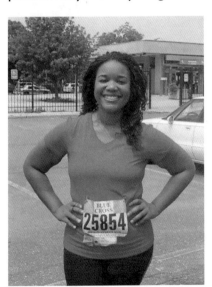

I was inspired to participate in more races after my first 5k. On the left is me after finishing The Broad Street Run (a ten-mile race).

Before I would feel like giving up when I failed to achieve outstanding results from week to week. But I had to remind myself that it's the small wins over time that build into greater victories. Each time I went to the gym when I didn't feel like it, or refused to binge on junk food at one o'clock in the morning, I knew I had accomplished something. And it's the same for you. No matter how you feel, you have to imagine yourself victorious in every moment. You're a winner at the starting line.

Chapter 4

Acceptance

Summer 2004

By the time I finished school, I had lost forty pounds and was feeling pretty good about myself. Although I picked up some weight since my lowest point at the time, I was happy to be smaller than I was before—a size eighteen instead of a size twenty-four. That's the cool thing about getting healthy; although it may be hard to get started and stick to it, the results make it all worth the effort. With my new stamina, confidence, and slimmer body, I knew I could take on the world....and taking on the world was just what I was about to do.

Here I was, only a few days after graduating from college, and traveling to West Africa with one of my closest friends. I had always wanted to go there, and having heard so many wonderful things about the people, food, music and cultures, I promised myself that one day I would. Well, the door opened and I was heading to the Motherland—Africa! We arrived first in Senegal and later hopped in the backseat of a crowded station wagon packed with strangers en route to our final destination, The Gambia.

I pressed my face against the window as the plane touched down so I could see the beautiful outline of the Continent—hues of blue and white waves crashing alongside the greenish-brown coastline. It was a beautiful site to see! My friend's study abroad host parents greeted us with a "Bonjour!" and embraced us with love and excitement. They were so happy to see us, and I was equally happy to see them.

As we waited for our car, the taxi cab drivers and airport workers greeted us with "Hello, my sister" and other such phrases. *My sister?* You will *never* hear that at the Philadelphia airport! Fortunately, the "Terranga," or welcoming culture, of Senegal accompanied us throughout the entire trip. We met with friends and family, ate lots of mangoes, drank orange Fanta, and dined on traditional West African dishes until we had our fill. We laughed hysterically, partied, toured, and relaxed our way through Senegal and The Gambia for two weeks. While in Africa, I truly felt free.

On one of our final evenings, a bunch of my new friends came to see me off. We sat in the courtyard and laughed, recapping stories of our trip and taking lots of pictures for memories. In that moment, my friend noticed something. "LeeAnn, you look so happy!" she said with the cheesiest grin you can imagine.

I chuckled and told her she was being overly sentimental, but she was right. For the first time in awhile, I stopped thinking about my weight. I fit in.

When I think back to how comfortable and free I felt, I admit I am a little surprised, given the circumstances. You see, during our trip people were not afraid to comment on my weight. In fact, it was probably talked about much more there than in the States. And nobody was safe. At the risk of making a broad generalization, most of the people we met were not afraid to comment on anybody's weight—fat or skinny.

I remember an incident in particular. One evening a family friend picked us up from our hotel for a night on the town. From then on he could not stop commenting on how much he liked "big" women like me. He said that we are healthy and not just skin and bones. (Pause: Let me be real for a second. In the States, if a guy said something like that to me, I would have to slap him. This guy only got away with it because he had a cool accent and was taking us out for the night. But dude, seriously?). Instead of getting offended, I laughed it off and went on my way. But it didn't stop there. Other men also found me physically attractive; my friend's host-brother, for example, fell in love with me during my stay and did not want to leave my side. Thankfully, he didn't comment on my weight, but I was still not used to being on the receiving end of all this male attention. For the first time *I* was the one the guys liked, and surprisingly, my "skinny" friend was getting much less attention than I was. At any rate, the more this continued, the more comfortable I felt in my own skin.

Don't get me wrong, this freedom to discuss weight didn't come without its uncomfortable moments. The little sister of a family friend hung out with us one day. She was sweet, ridiculously curious, and like any other teenage girl, boy crazy. During our visit to the local market place, she asked me a simple question: "Don't you want to lose weight and be skinny?" Naturally, I was tempted to teach her some manners, but I noticed innocence in her eyes and in the tone of her voice. Good question, I guess. Were our Western ideals of beauty and femininity influencing this culture? This can't be a good thing, can it?

At home, being "bigger" was associated with so many negative things—you can be smart, but not hot; you can be friendly, but not flirty; you can have a great personality, but you definitely can't be an airhead if you don't have a perfect body. In West Africa it meant something completely different. Actually, it had no meaning at all— being "bigger" meant you were just...bigger. It did not make you good or bad. There, my weight was more of a fact than an issue—it was not *my* weight. It was not me.

I left Africa with a new sense of self. I wasn't wildly more confident or self-accepting, but I was just a bit more content. In the first few days back in the States I took some risks on love, spoke out more, and cared less about how I looked all the time.

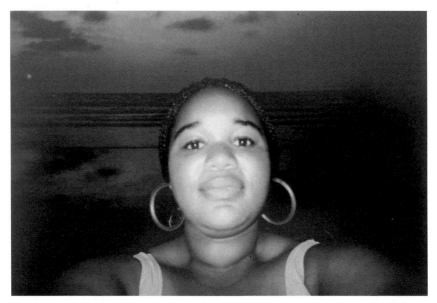

This is the beautiful sunset at a beach in The Gambia—breathtaking.

I wish that sense of being lingered a bit longer than it did. Either way, my idea of who I was began to shift some more, and this time in the right direction.

My two-week stay helped in so many other ways as well. For one, it encouraged me to stop measuring myself against women that were half my size. What is considered beauty in the West was something completely different in other parts of the world. This *This trip also taught* trip also taught me that my weight did not *me that my weight* have to be a qualifying factor used to measure *did not have to be* my worth. And yeah okay, the attention from *a qualifying factor* the men didn't hurt either! *used to measure* Although getting special treatment *my worth.* from the guys was an added plus, there was something greater taking place. What was developing was a passion for a healthier me. I didn't realize this transformation was happening, but going to Africa was an awesome experience that opened my eyes to how beautiful I really was, size eight, eighteen, or twenty-four.

In your own journey to lose weight and regain your health, don't discount the little things to help boost your confidence. Now you may not call a trip to Africa a "little thing," but having fun and getting the attention I had never experienced at home were small moments that motivated me. And soon something wonderful soon began to take shape. For the first time I started to love my body like I never had before. Instead of feeling ashamed about my size, I began to feel like a new woman. A woman that was ready to step out and conquer the world.

I didn't quite realize it at the time, but a big burden was gradually lifting as I continued to accept myself just the way I was. Now granted, I didn't use this confidence level to eat whatever I wanted and remain obese. But rather, it gave me the courage to accept myself as I was and love myself enough to better my habits. Furthermore, I placed less emphasis on others' opinions, as I came to a greater understanding of myself. It was becoming more and more apparent that weight is something you can lose or gain at any time. But having a beautiful, peaceful spirit, and self-confidence is far more important.

True self-acceptance means loving and liking yourself, regardless of how much you weigh. As I'm sure you know, this is easier said than done. Before I stepped out on my weight loss journey, I constantly struggled with accepting myself as the 289-pound girl. I guess it was good that I had hoop dreams of being thin and healthy, but this quickly turned into a subconscious hatred of things I could and could not change about me. After losing the weight and reaching my ultimate goal I realized something—I still felt the same. For about a year after reaching my lowest point, I still felt uncomfortable in my clothes, I still thought I looked fat in certain outfits, and I was surprised and even disappointed when my six-pack abs didn't magically appear. Hoop dreams.

From a size twenty-four to six, I have seen life from the perspective of ten different women. I know the embarrassment of having to exit a roller coaster ride after the attendant couldn't buckle me into the seat. On the other hand, I also know the extreme satisfaction of asking the salesperson to exchange a dress for the next size down. I have been the average size, the smaller size, and the plus size during my short time on this earth. Without a doubt the hardest lesson I learned was that no matter what the size of my skirt is, the insecurities do not just fade away.

I know this may sound silly to you, but even as a little girl in the fifth grade, I believed that with the perfect body would come the perfect life. Once I reached my goals, I thought I would be satisfied. I'd have the courage to pursue my acting career, and then of course find love and live happily ever after. It all seemed like a natural progression: weight loss, professional success, marriage, white picket fence, two and a half kids, and a dog named Spot. You get the picture.

I guess you can't blame me for believing such a lie since everything around us tells us that this message is true. Every television sitcom, movie, and music video confirms this "fact" as reality. The illusion is that being thin and pretty equals happiness. The funny thing is, I was already living a great life. I had a family who loved me, was educated in some of the country's finest schools and universities, and had more friends than I could count. To top it off, I also had a relationship with God that made me feel secure and gave me an optimistic view that all things in life work together for the good. Yet, I still believed that something was missing. Unfortunately, no matter how much weight I lost, and no matter how "good" I looked, I still wanted more. I was not content.

Acceptance became a journey of its own. After being just about every size in the Ladies' section at Macy's, I came to the conclusion that this dissatisfaction had to stop. I'm not sure exactly when this epiphany occurred (and maybe it's still happening), but one day I realized that I had to just believe I was okay *today*. Yes, I wanted to achieve my weight loss goals and be healthy, but I did not want to torture myself along the way.

I've learned that in order to *feel* successful I must be content. Contentment for me comes with appreciating each stage that I'm in. Through my weight loss experience, I discovered that I was strong, had courage, and a lot of heart—even at 289 pounds. You see, success is incremental and may not always show up on the scale. While working towards my weight loss goals, I trained with a professional athlete, tried hip hop dancing for the first time, and even completed a ten-mile race. I also ventured out in my professional, educational, and love life. I did not discover a bikini-wearing hot girl after losing weight. I discovered *me*.

> *I did not discover a bikini-wearing hot girl after losing weight. I discovered me.*

However, before this discovery I used to beat myself up when I didn't feel strong or when I fell off the wagon. Now, I try to remind myself that it's okay to make mistakes and there's always tomorrow, or even the next meal. Forgiveness, especially forgiving yourself, is such a critical part to losing weight. You have to let yourself off the hook because you won't do everything perfectly all the time. The more you do this, the more willing you are to continue on your journey even when you fall. We're all working on some things, but let's accept the fact that we are fabulous today. If nothing changes or if it all changes, you are still a D.I.V.A.

****

Here's a poem God gave me to learn the lesson of acceptance. I hope it encourages you to do the same:

Who's the Treasure?
I'm the Treasure
Who's the Treasure?
Me
I am the Treasure
This call and response is a little something my Heavenly Father gave to me
When I was feeling down, uncute, and unwanted He told me who He
    declared me to be
He told me to not be so concerned about who others say that I am
And He most certainly told me not to be concerned about whether or not
    I got a man
Or more money, or that new job, or whether or not I have the perfect body
See I'm learning to love myself
Big hips, big thighs, loud laugh and even those jokes that only I think are
    funny
Yes, I am the Treasure
I'm the Bentley with the diamond encrusted spinnin' rims
I'm those new PZI jeans that only us curvaceous women can fit in
Yes, I'm high class
I'm your Versace, your Louis, and for those of you who want to throw it back
I am all of that and the bag of chips, with the dip, and the chicken noodle
    soup and the soda on the side
I told you I'm the Treasure
I'm the one who attracts those "Ay Yurps" and the "Cssts" and the
    "Shortay's" as I walk down the street
But you best believe I'm also that girl who knows how to worship at Jesus'
    feet
I'm a business woman, an entertainer, I'm that Proverbs 31 woman that
    the Bible talks about
I'm worth so much that even in my imperfections I deserve some clout

I am the Treasure
I'm the "Sought After" one as it describes in Isaiah 62 and 12
I'm the holy temple wherein the Spirit of God Himself dwells
No, I'm not claiming to be the "every" woman that Whitney Houston and
    Chaka Khan sang so beautifully to be
I'm just sayin' I'm that "more-than-enough-anointed" woman that will
    help a brotha birth his destiny
Yes, I am the Treasure,
Because the Treasure lives on the inside of me
I'm the Treasure because that's who my Daddy proclaimed me to be
I am the Treasure,
And girlfriend you should know what you are too
See we were all created in His image, so just relax and let Him do what
    He do
Like Ray Charles, we should be blind or should I say deaf to what the
    world has to say
Because all those opinions of the naysayers are not going to matter at the
    end of the day
Because
You are the Treasure
Scream it, purr it, or even shout!
You are the one that God can't stop thinking about
Daily, He refreshes, every moment He renews
He wants to be your Advocate, your Counselor, and yes He evens wants
    to be your boo
So the next time you think about chasing, stalking, or seeking after any man
Consider God, the Great Romancer
Tell me, who can love you better than He can

Conclusion

So, where am I now? At this point I've realized that there is no set destination to total health and wellness—it is a journey that continues for a lifetime. I have recommitted to working on my weight loss slowly with an emphasis on establishing healthy habits. Instead of only focusing on the scale, it is now my new norm to workout regularly, watch my sugar intake, and yes, even eat more broccoli! The pounds may not be dropping as quickly as before when I was on stricter programs, but I know this type of weight loss will last. I still cringe at times when I think that "this" will never end.

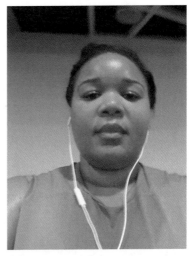

Sweaty after a cardio session while out of town on business. I constantly remind myself that this is a lifestyle for me now, not just a diet.

Yet, I am comforted with the understanding that we should always strive to get better. There's no stopping when it comes to becoming healthier—we should always be working towards that.

As I reflect on my journey, I am certain that it takes discipline, inspiration, walking in victory, and self-acceptance to be and feel successful. I've found this to be true in any area of my life. I sometimes laugh now at how overzealous I was when I first started to write this book. I had just lost a ton of weight and wanted to share my success with the world, one chunky person at a time. Now that *I* am the one who's in need of help, I have to challenge myself to adopt the same principles I intended to share with others.

Does this really work? Are these really the keys to success? My heart and my mind resoundingly say, "yes."

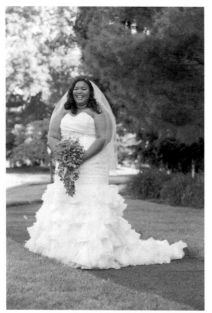

That's me on my wedding day on June 7, 2014. I learned that I do not have to wait to be thin to experience happiness. I can enjoy my life as I strive for my goals.

For where I am right now, I especially need inspiration and self-acceptance more than ever. When I was at my goal weight I wrote a comment in my journal that still challenges me today: "Even if I gain all the weight back, I know I can lose it again with the confidence and principles I've learned through this process." That was such a bold statement. Back then I felt so confident in the strength I demonstrated to myself that I believed I could do it all over again if I had to. Looking back, I'm desperately pulling on that confidence, because I honestly don't feel it as strongly as I did before. I have doubts that I can or even want to go through the weight loss process again. But, I have to believe that I can. I don't have to *feel* like I can do it to be successful. I just have to believe.

If there is anything that you should take away from my story, please understand that with or without the extra pounds you are beautiful. You are strong. Full of life. Capable of anything. And with God anything is possible. All of my life, I dreamed of being thin. Now that I have experienced it, I realize that being a D.I.V.A. is so much sweeter.

Appendix

DIVA TIPS

Discipline

1. Discipline is not self-hatred.
2. Discipline takes practice.
3. Be willing to wait for what you want.
4. Discipline is a physical, mental and spiritual thing.

Inspiration

1. Keep your vision in mind.
2. Be willing to redefine and adjust your goals.
3. Inspiration drives out fear and strengthens your faith.
4. Inspiration comes from God.

Victory

1. Get started now.
2. Get out of your comfort zone.
3. Find your personal rhythm.
4. See yourself as a winner now.

Acceptance

1. Find something to love about yourself today.
2. Exchange negative thoughts with positive words.
3. Decide to enjoy your life.

MORE THOUGHTS ON DISCIPLINE

Developing discipline, just like losing weight, is definitely a step-by-step process. And don't be fooled into focusing simply on the calories and food choices. I've learned that physical discipline alone does not necessarily bring complete success. Discipline, as I've come to understand it during my ten-year weight loss journey, has many faces: physical, mental, and spiritual. In the early stages of my weight loss, I was fixated on exercise, calorie-cutting, and portion control. It's true that physical discipline helped me get through intense cardio workouts on the elliptical and replace meals with diet shakes. However, as I progressed on my journey, I came to understand the importance of mental and spiritual discipline as well. Today I still lean on mental discipline to get my body out of the bed at 5 a.m. to workout or to say "no" to the temptation of eating fattening foods. Through spiritual discipline I have found the confidence and inner strength to press forward. At times when I'm feeling defeated, I depend on prayer, meditation on positive affirmations, and scriptural promises to keep me going. I also make it a point to surround myself with optimistic people that encourage me and challenge me to do my best. Endurance and sustained success come when all three forms of discipline are working together at the same time.

I experienced this firsthand during the family reunion weekend in 2001. Although I had exercised physical discipline throughout that first day, I knew I did not have enough mental discipline to turn down the buffet. Temptation was everywhere! So I did what any other respectable soldier would do, I retreated! Yet, after doing so, I felt like I made the wrong choice. Thoughts of failure, embarrassment, and shame flooded my mind as I sat in the motel room all alone. I was mentally exhausted. But after moments of moping around in self-pity, something happened. I began to draw on the positive deposits that had been made in my heart through practicing spiritual discipline. In that moment my heart reminded me of the prayers I had prayed, the goals I had envisioned, and the past successes I had experienced. And I *knew* that I was not a failure. When my body and mind failed me, my heart (or spirit) did the work. Physical, mental and spiritual discipline is critical to weight loss success. Spiritual discipline, however, acts as the true catalyst for motivation and change. You may experience momentary success without it, but with it, you will lay a foundation that will sustain you through every leg of the journey.

In a nutshell, start to look at discipline as self-love and not self-hate. Being disciplined means you have control over circumstances like overeating rather than the circumstances having power or control over you. Discipline helps you to achieve your goals, not keep you from them. Begin to see discipline as something just as important to master during your weight loss journey as avoiding processed sugar food items. It's that important. Becoming more disciplined with what I eat and consistently working out wasn't easy, but I did it and so can you!

TIPS FROM THE TRAINER

From *The Play Book by Coach Chuck*

So often people believe that only a select few have the discipline that is required to start and maintain a fitness program. And that is just not the case. We all have the ability within us to apply the discipline needed to reach our fitness goals. I like to call it the three P's: patience, practice and push-through.

You have to exercise *patience* when setting your health and fitness goals. One of the most important things to do is set realistic goals that have proper allotments of time, while also accounting for the unforeseen obstacles of life. Even though you see advertisement campaigns that talk about great weight loss changes in just twelve weeks, you need to disregard the "quick fix" thinking that promises you unbelievable results with minimal effort. In fact, most people would be surprised to find out that losing two pounds a week is considered a very successful program.

Secondly, you have to *practice* positive thoughts and goal-oriented actions everyday. These will support a healthier you and motivate you along your journey. Realize that it won't happen over night, though, so you don't need to get down on yourself because you ate an entire bowl of ice cream or because you quit halfway into your training session. The reason it's called practice is because you have not totally changed your life from the bad habits of the past. *Webster's* says a practitioner is "one who does anything customary or habitual." For the most part diets don't work because your brain associates it with the negative, like the tearing away from something you used to enjoy. As you replace bad choices with good ones, remind yourself that you're still learning to keep healthy habits. You're not just finding out how to play the game, but to master it.

One of the best ways for you to fuel your body successfully is to adopt "Best Choice Eating." In order to do so, commit to the following two things:

1. Make the decision that from this day forward you *are* a healthy eater.
2. Decide that you want to make the best food choice available in any and every situation. Start by just picking one thing at a time to change, i.e., drink eight glasses of water for two weeks, and in the next two weeks add on to that goal.

The last factor in reaching your fitness goals requires you to *push through* all the issues and past excuses that would hold you back. You may not be able to go 100mph all the time and the roads will get rough, but just keep pushing forward. However slow the progress may seem on the outside, it is still progress if you continue to move forward. For instance, one of LeeAnn's initial goals was to exercise five times a week. Instead of starting with five days right away, she committed to gradually increasing her commitment week by week until she reached her goal. The point is, you have to allow yourself to go at your own pace.

These three P's of patience, practice, and push-through will help you develop and maintain a healthier and more active lifestyle that will work for you.

****

COACH CHUCK'S TIPS IN ACTION

Apply these practical tips to your daily routine, and you will lose weight and also become a healthier, more energetic you.

On Nutrition:

- Drink eight glasses of water a day. Avoid drinking soda.
- Have dairy only once a day.
- Eat three meals a day with a light snack in between.
- Refrain from carbohydrates four hours before you go to bed.
- Try eating a fruit and vegetable diet two days a week.

On Fitness:
<u>A Four Week Plan</u>

Week One:

- Get started with just ten minutes a day.
- Stretch five minutes.
- Complete the following rotation:
  o 10 squats
  o 10 pushups
  o 10 leg lifts
  o 45-second break
- Repeat this as many times as you can for five minutes.

Week Two:

- Repeat week one exercises.

Week Three:

- Stretch five minutes.
- Double the amount of each activity from the last two weeks.
- Complete the following rotation:
  o 20 squats
  o 20 pushups
  o 20 leg lifts
  o Add a plank hold for 30 seconds to the rotation.
  o 45-second break

Week Four:

- Stretch five minutes.

- **Complete the following rotation two times:**
  - o 20 squats
  - o 20 pushups
  - o 20 leg lifts
  - o 30-second plank hold
- Take a **45**-second break every two rotations.
- Repeat this as many times as you can for twenty minutes.

* Want to take it to the next level? Complete this rotation as many times as you can:

- 30 seconds of running in place
- 45 seconds of squats
- 45 seconds of pushups
- 45 seconds of leg lifts
- 45-second plank hold

On Healthy Habits:

- Plan your food a day in advance: For example, try bringing your lunch to work. Or, if you're going out to lunch, find a restaurant with healthy choices and look up the menu ahead of time.
- Don't skip meals—it won't help you to lose weight: Remember your body is a machine so it needs good fuel.
- Measure success in other ways: The scale is only a fraction of a much larger equation and shouldn't be used as the only gauge to success. Instead of depending solely on the scale, pick a pair of jeans or an outfit that you'd like to fit better and use that as your measuring tape. It's definitely more fun than the scale!

- Think deeply about your goals: When you set them, ask yourself, *Where did these come from?*—Are these goals your own, or have they been put on you by others?
- Set smaller, attainable goals: Set a major goal that you would like to meet at the end of six months. Then choose three concrete steps to help get you there. As you complete each step, celebrate with something other than food.
- Make a note of it: At the end of each day, write down some things that you did well and some things that you'd like to do better the next day. This will put an end to the day and help you sleep better.
- Get around positive people: Distance yourself from negative people until you are strong enough to impact them and not the other way around. Sharing your dreams and goals with people who motivate you will help you achieve greater success.
- Get your mind right: Each night take time to read inspirational books, articles, or scriptures, and focus on suggestions on healthy living and the success stories of others. Doing so will help you glean enough inspiration to make it through the next day.

For more tips from Coach Chuck visit:
http://chuckmorrisfitness.com

LEEANN'S GO-TO RECIPES

Go-to-Mains

Broiled Chicken Wings

Ingredients:

- Whole Chicken Wings
- Extra Virgin Olive Oil
- Onion Powder
- Creole Seasoning
- Crushed Red Pepper Seeds
- Broiler Pan

Preparation:

1. Pre-heat oven to Broil or to bake at 450 degrees
2. Rinse chicken wings with water and place on broiler pan
3. Very lightly drizzle each wing with Olive Oil (Olive Oil Cooking Spray works well too)
4. Sprinkle a generous amount of onion powder and crushed red pepper seeds on both sides of the wings. Sprinkle sparingly creole seasoning on the wings (too much will make it salty)
5. Place uncovered into the pre-heated oven and cook for about 20 minutes, then turn to other side
6. Complete cooking on opposite side for another 10 – 15 minutes or until the skin is nice and crisp

*Watch your portions. One or two wings is just enough.

Baked Tilapia

Ingredients:

- Fresh or frozen Tilapia filets (I purchase the large bag of frozen filets available at most grocery stores)
- Extra Virgin Olive Oil (or Olive Oil cooking spray)
- Creole Seasoning
- Dried Parsley
- Paprika for color

Instructions:

1. Pre-heat oven to bake at 350 degrees
2. Place thawed fish filets on a baking sheet lined with non-stick aluminum foil (easier to clean!)
3. Very lightly drizzle the fish with Olive Oil (Olive Oil Cooking Spray works well too)
4. Sprinkle a generous amount of Parsley, Crushed Red Pepper Seeds, and Paprika onto the fish. Sprinkle sparingly Creole Seasoning on the fish (too much will make it salty).
5. Add a small amount of water just enough to cover the bottom of the baking sheet for moisture
6. Place uncovered into the pre-heated oven and cook for about 20 - 25 minutes or until the fish is flaky when cut with a fork

*For additional flavor, cut a half of a medium white onion into thin slices and layer on top of the fish filets before baking.

Grilled Chicken

Ingredients:

- Boneless chicken breasts
- Extra Virgin Olive Oil (or Olive Oil cooking spray)
- Creole Seasoning
- Dried Parsley
- Garlic powder

Instructions:

1. Very lightly drizzle the chicken breasts with Olive Oil (Olive Oil Cooking Spray works well too)
2. Season chicken breast generously with seasonings
3. Pre-heat a grill pan on the stovetop (a grill pan will give the chicken those lovely grill marks)
4. When the pan is very hot, place chicken breasts on grill pan.
5. Cook for 5 minutes on each side until cooked thoroughly.

Go-to Sides

Steamed Broccoli

Ingredients:

- A couple heads of Broccoli Florets
- Water
- Teaspoon of butter
- Salt and Pepper to taste

Preparation:

1. Cut Broccoli Florets off the head to make individual florets

2. Rinse in colander
3. Place in a microwave safe bowl
4. Add water to cover the bottom of bowl (roughly 1 inch deep)
5. Cover with plastic wrap or a microwave safe top
6. Cook on high for 3 or 4 minutes or until tender with a bit of crunch
7. Toss with the butter and salt and pepper to taste

(Healthier cooking option is to steam the broccoli stove-top in a steamer basket in a pot).

Steamed Green Beans

Follow the same instructions as with the Steamed Broccoli. Or, purchase fresh Green Beans pre-packaged in a steamer bag and place in the microwave for a few minutes. This can usually be found in the fresh produce section of the grocery store.

Steamed Brown Rice

Ingredients:

- Instant "boil in the bag" rice
- Water

Preparation:

Simply follow the instructions on the box! If you must know, fill a medium sauce pan about 3 quarters full of water. Place the individual "boil in the bag" of rice into the pan. Boil on high for about 12 – 15 minutes. Cut open the bag and pour into your serving dish.

Roasted Potatoes

Ingredients:

- 3 - 4 white potatoes (or sweet potatoes for extra nutrition and flavor)
- Extra Virgin Olive Oil
- Crushed Red Pepper
- Thyme
- Rosemary
- Black Pepper
- Salt to taste

Instructions:

1. Pre-heat oven to bake at 450 degrees
2. Cut potatoes with skin on into square or triangle pieces (roughly an inch in diameter). Set aside in cold water
3. In a small bowl, add an 1/8 cup Olive Oil
4. In the same bowl, add about a tablespoon each of the seasons (except the salt) to the Olive Oil. Add a half teaspoon of salt. Mix ingredients.
5. Toss the potatoes in the Olive Oil mixture until fully covered
6. Place the potatoes onto a baking sheet in a single layer
7. Bake for 30 – 40 minutes or until tender. I prefer my potatoes a tad crisp!

Go-to Sweet Endings

Banana Ice Cream

Ingredients:

- 2 – 4 bananas sliced
- Cup of frozen berries or other frozen fruit as desired

Instructions:

1. At least 2 hours prior, peel and then slice bananas into coin-sized pieces. Put into a freezer bag and place in the freezer for up to 2 hours or until frozen.
2. In a food processor or a good blender, chop the frozen bananas using a light pulse until a creamy consistency forms (chopping on high may create heat and melt the bananas)
3. Add other frozen fruit to taste as desired such as frozen strawberries
4. Scoop and eat immediately

Other Go-to Sweet Endings

- Sugar-free Jello and light whipped cream (I prefer RediWhip)
- Sliced apple with a tablespoon of peanut butter
- Bowl of blueberries and sliced strawberries with light whipped cream to top